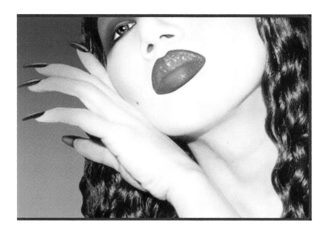

Do It Yourself Acrylic Nails with Acrylic Nail Art
© 2012, Virginia Reali

GW00537602

PREFACE

I started in the nail supply industry in the late 1990's. I was desperate to get some supplies for my nail art hobby and they were not available in Australia, so I had to import them. I realised that if I was after these products then there must be others who would like to buy these products in Australia and from there BMNE Direct started. Very quickly we filled a large gap in the nail supply industry offering our customers anything and everything we could find for nail art.

Our business quickly expanded to cover all aspects of artificial nails and we learnt how to use each of the products we sold. With experienced nail technicians working with us it is great fun to experiment, play and develop new products. We attended specialty classes and Expos finding new products and expanding our knowledge of the industry.

We found that people would purchase an acrylic kit but stumble when things went wrong and this book hopefully will help the budding nail artist overcome those stumbling blocks and enable them to create gorgeous acrylic nails and have a play with some nail art.

Virginia Reali

TABLE OF CONTENTS

Chapter 1

GETTING STARTED

Learning to do your own acrylic nails is easy. It will save you time and money. This book is a guide presented in layperson's terms with step by step with illustrations.

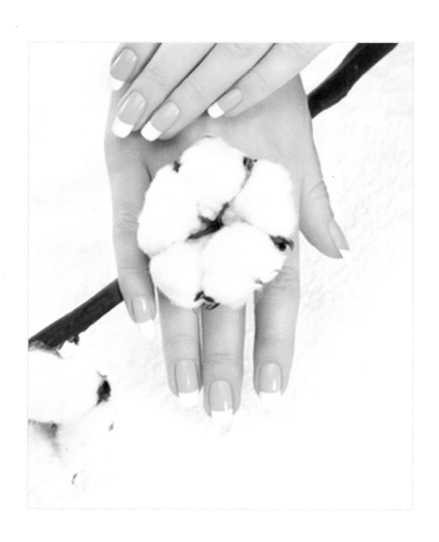

Section 1

Why do your own nails

1. Nails Salons

2. Doing it yourself

3. Equipment

4. Acrylic Kits

Chances are you have been wearing acrylic nails for sometime and now wanting to your own nails at home. Maybe you want to learn how to do acrylic nails on yourself and your friends.

While this book is about you applying your own acrylic nails, I believe it is important to have a little background knowledge on the industry.

NAIL SALONS

They seem to pop up everywhere and there are always people in them getting their nails done or having a manicure or pedicure. The cost for a full set of nails with acrylic varies from shop to shop and country to country. In recent times there have been many news reports of customers who have gone to a nail bar, had their nails done and ended up with a major fungal infection which usually renders their nails unable to have any application of either acrylic or gel applied again because the infections are so damaging and prolonged. Sadly we are able to generalise about these nail bars in that they have no hygiene standards, the products they use are inferior and in some cases illegal, the operators have a poor grasp of your countries native language and little or no training. The price of a full set of nails at these types of nail bars is usually a lot cheaper than that of a nail bar which is run by staff that have completed a formal course offering qualifications.

At a salon that charges a higher price, you will usually get far better service and personal attention, there is no queue out the door (that is not because they charge more, it is because they schedule their clients effectively), they use quality products, their salons are clean, welcoming and relaxing, their staff have all been trained by professionals or have attended a nail tech school and they use good quality professional products and hygiene is usually at the top of their to do list. For these important extras I would not hesitate in paying extra. Sadly because people are often unaware of what can await them in a cheap nail bar they attend there and the nail bar owned and operated by staff who have qualifications ends up going out of business because they are unable to compete with the cheap prices.

There are many manufacturers of acrylic products worldwide. One product, which is banned from being used with acrylic nails, is MMA (METHYL METHACRYLATE). It is banned because it is a health risk (Google MMA to read about the health risks associated with MMA). This ban applies to USA and in Australia no more that 1% of MMA can be used in the liquid used with acrylic powder and this is acrylic monomer. Acrylic Monomer containing MMA is still manufactured and it is used in the dental industry because of its strength in dentures. Acrylic Monomer containing MMA is cheap in comparison to an EMA (Ethyl Methacrylate) Acrylic Monomer. EMA Monomer has been deemed to be a lot safer for use in acrylic nails. Both monomers smell but an MMA monomer has a stronger and sickly sweet smell that lingers whereas an EMA monomer smell is not so sickly sweet and dissipates within a minute. MMA monomer sets like concrete, it cannot be soaked off and has to be filed off by hand or drilled right down to a thin layer then hand filed off. MMA monomer will damage your nail plate, making the natural nail soft and discoloured. Also, if you knock your nails when you are wearing MMA based acrylic nails you run the risk of ripping your entire nail from the nail bed.

DOING IT YOURSELF

By doing your own nails at home you will eliminate or hugely minimise the risk of fungal infections, you will save money and you will be able to do your nails in your own time. You might think it looks too hard but it isn't, all it takes is a little practice to get it right.

EQUIPMENT

1. A well ventilated warm room - the ventilation is needed because of the fumes from the monomer, they can, to some, seem very strong. A little bit of warmth helps with the products drying.

2. A table that you can rest your arm on as you are doing each hand and has plenty of room to spread your products out on.

3. Protection for the table is advised because if you spill any of the products onto the table they may damage the surface. Paper towels are excellent, put down two to three layers. A towel under the paper towels is also a good idea.

4. A comfortable chair at the table so that you feel relaxed when doing your nails.

5. A kit containing good quality products.

WHAT SHOULD YOUR ACRYLIC KIT CONTAIN?

Some of the larger retails stores sell small kits for doing acrylic nails but these are designed to do one set and will not last past a few days before they fall off or lifting starts.

A good kit should have:

- at least 100 nail tips in assorted sizes
- A Kolinsky hair acrylic brush for application
- Acrylic powder
- EMA acrylic monomer
- Anti Bacterial Solution
- Tip cutters
- Glass dappen
- Foam files for filing the acrylic

- Whiteblock
- 3 way buffing block
- Cuticle sticks
- Primer
- Nail Prep
- Cuticle Oil
- Top coat
- Glue for adhering tips to your nails.
- A brush for dusting away filing dust from nails.

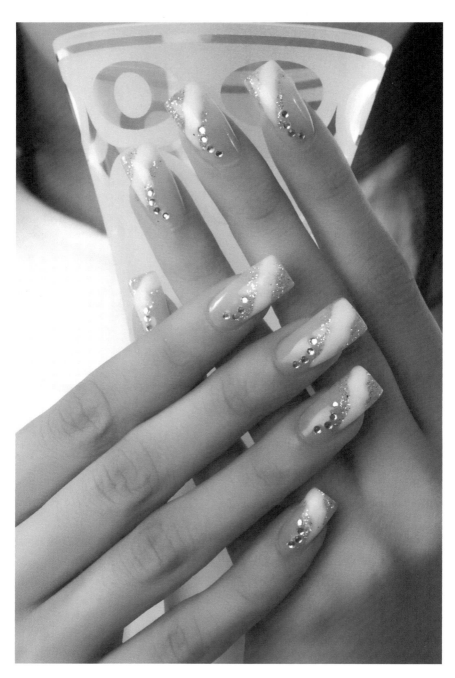

Create this look using the reverse technique and instead of doing a smile line, finish on an angle and then butt up white to your first application of clear, and then butt up silver glitter acrylic to that. Use clear tips.

Section 2

EVERYTHING IN YOUR KIT

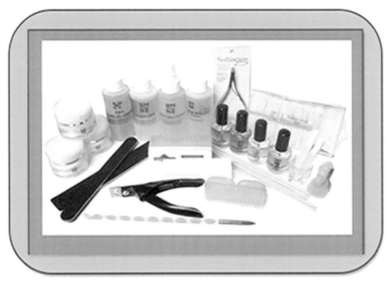

A brief description of what the items in your kit are used for and what they contain.

1. Acrylic Monomer - ensure that it is an EMA monomer, if you are unsure contact the seller and ask.

2. Acrylic Powders - in a good quality kit there should be three different colour powders, clear, pink and white. The pink should be a translucent pink, the clear should be crystal clear (clear powder will appear white in the container) and the white should be a bright white.

3. Anti-Bacterial Solution is a necessity, this will assist in stopping fungal infections and keep your equipment bacteria free.

4. Nail Prep is used to remove natural oils from the nail plate, this will keep the nail plate oil free for about 30 minutes.

5. Primer is one of the most important components in the application process. Primer is an acid and it sets down a chemical base for your acrylic to adhere to. There are two types of primers available on the market one is acid based and one is a non-acid based primer for sensitive skin.

6. Cuticle Oil is used when you have finished.

7. Either a round or oval acrylic brush is suitable, make sure there are no fly away bristles, if there is one or two trim them back with nail scissors. The brush size should be either an 8 or 10, anything larger is too large and anything smaller will not give you an even finish.

8. A glass dappen is used for the acrylic monomer, you pour as much as you need for one full application of 10 fingers into the dappen. It is a very small glass cup.

9. Tip cutters are for trimming the tips after you have glued them onto your natural nails. There are three different positions you can hold the cutters to get different cuts. The first position \ will cut a well into a tip before it is applied to the nail, use this to take full well tips to 1/2 well tips. The position | will give you a straight square cut and the third position of / will give a slightly rounded edge.

10. White blocks are used for gently removing the shine from the natural nails before starting and smoothing over the acrylic application when you have finished.

11. The 3 way shiner block is used after the whiteblock, when you have finished and this will remove any surface cuts from filing the acrylic application, it can also be used to add a shine to the application

12. The files in your kit should be foam files with a mix of grits between 100 and 180. The lower the grit number the coarser the grit. These files are used for removing overhangs of acrylic on the free edge and if you have raised areas in your application these files will bring them down quickly. These files are also used for removing the acrylic (more on that later).

13. Glue - always keep the lid on your glue when it is not in use.

14. Cuticle sticks are helpful for removing the acrylic off the cuticle area before it dries.

15. Soak Off/Acetone is used for soaking acrylic nails off.

16. Dusting brush is used to brush away dust and excess material from the nails before application.

NAIL TIPS

There are several different types of nail tips available.

- Full well - used for nails that have been bitten, these tips give more cover and strength over the natural nail area.

- 1/2 well - the well at the end of the tip is butted up against the natural nail free edge and the well is glued to the natural nail.

- French white - always comes with a 1/2 well but are available with many different types of smile line.

- Tips are available in Natural, White and Clear as well as airbrushed or tips with designs already embedded into the tip and coloured tips.

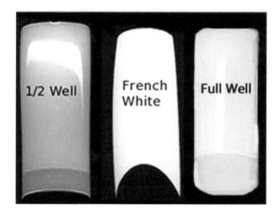

Tips also come in a variety of colours and are great for a different French nail finish.

ABOUT ACRYLIC POWDER AND ACRYLIC MONOMER

Your acrylic application consists of two parts - the powder and the liquid monomer. When you are using the monomer, pour as much as you need into the glass dappen, do not tip your brush into your bottle because if you have powder on your brush you will contaminate the liquid and it will start to thicken. When you have finished your application do not pour any leftover monomer back into the bottle because the liquid in the dappen will have traces of powder. Get an absorbent paper towel, scrunch it up and push it into the dappen to soak up the excess liquid then put this paper towel into a sealable plastic bag and dispose of it.

When you first start you will need to play with the powder and monomer to get a good consistency ratio between the two products. A mix that is too wet will take too long to set and have no strength and will peel. A mix that is too dry will also be weak and not set properly. Grab a couple of tips and practice. A good mix will set within a minute, it will be smooth and you will feel it warming up slightly as it starts to set. To check to see if it has set, get a cuticle stick or the top part of the handle of your brush and tap gently on the application, if it sounds hollow then it is set.

YOUR BRUSH

Before you start you need to condition your brush, do this by dipping all the bristles into monomer, wipe the brush on the edge of the dappen and then wipe it over a paper towel, repeat this process a couple of times. This is done to make the bristles ready to hold the liquid, the bristles on the brush take up the liquid and the liquid comes down through the bristles to moisten the bead of powder when you pick it up.

VARIETIES OF FRENCH NAIL TIPS

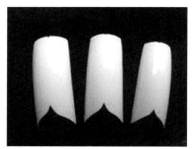 

Fancy V French   U shape or deep

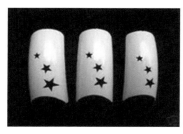

Star nails, put tape on the underneath of the tip and fill with coloured acrylic or glitter acrylic from the top, buff back to the tip. Also available are heart, daisy and small circle tips.

Clear Tips are generally used when doing specialty nail art where you want a slightly translucent finish and to be able to see the nail art underneath the tip as well.
Clear tips are available in ½ well (as pictured) or full well.

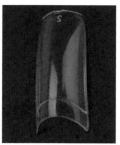

Chapter 2

FIRST STEPS

Each stage is crucial to ensure you apply a good application. Don't skip anything, if you do, things may not turn out so well.

Read through the entire book before you start, this will give you a better understanding of the entire process.

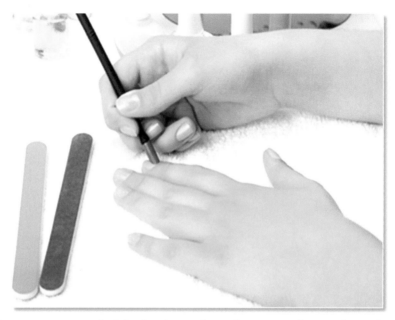

Use an orangewood stick, plastic cuticle pusher or stainless steel cuticle pusher to very gently push your cuticles back before starting. This is done to remove any excess cuticle so that when you apply the acrylic it is not sitting on any cuticle. If the acrylic sits on the cuticle you will get lifting and air pockets that could let an infection in. This is also why when applying the acrylic you need to make sure it is not touching your cuticle area because if it is it can create an air pocket. You need to ensure a solid adhesion to the nail plate to minimize any chance of lifting later.

Section 1

THE PREPARATION PROCESS

1. Other items you will need
2. Getting work area ready
3. Sizing and fitting tips
4. Preparing nail for tips
5. Pre acrylic applications and explanations

Set your table up and lay everything out so that it is in easy reach while you are sitting in your chair. Layout a towel on the table and then 2-3 layers of paper towel on top of that.

Using nail clippers, clip your natural nails back to line up with the edge of your finger or a little further back if can, leave enough room to butt a tip up against the tip.

Before you even sit down to start you will need to wash your hands thoroughly, preferably with an antibacterial hand wash. Give them a good scrub especially around the cuticles. Use a cuticle stick to gently push your cuticle back making sure there is no cuticle on the area you are going to apply acrylic.

If you have any bits of loose skin around the cuticles use a pair of nail scissors to trim these back. Do not pull them off.

You need to size your tips before the next step. Take a tip and hold it on a 45 degree angle against the free edge of your nail and then angle the tips well onto your nail. Does it fit neatly - not short on the sides of the tip to your nail and not overhanging the sides of your nail? Does it fit without having to push it onto the natural nail to make it meet the natural nail? If the answer is Yes, you have the right size. Do not try to force a tip onto the nail because it will lift off the nail shortly after you have glued it down. You need to have a snug fit onto the nail plate and the sides of the nail plate area against the cuticles without the tip touching the cuticles. If you have a tip that touches the sides of the nail but fits neatly onto the nail plate, grab a foam file and file the sides of the tip down until the sides of the tip no longer touch the cuticle when fitted to the nail, do this before gluing it onto the nail.

The tips you have should be sized from 0-9 or 1-10. Size each nail against a tip from the thumb to the smallest finger. Lay the tips out in front of you from largest to smallest and do two rows, one for each hand. Do not assume that the left hand sizing will be the same as the right hand. You will need to size up each individual finger.

Take a cuticle stick and GENTLY push back the cuticles and scrape away, carefully, any excess cuticle on the nail.

The next step is one of the most important steps. Spray your fingers with Antibacterial solution and let it dry thoroughly. The antibacterial is going to help eliminate any nasties that may be hiding on your fingers.

Now, take the white block and gently buff off the shine on your natural nail. This will also create a slightly rough surface, which will help give the acrylic a surface to adhere to. DO NOT buff and buff, a gentle buff down is all that is needed. Remember, you do not want to damage the top of your nail plate. Try not to hit your cuticles as well.

Use your dust brush and brush away all the filings, if you can't get them all off, run your hands under water, dry and spray again with Antibacterial solution and let it dry.

Grab your glass dappen and your glue. Open your glue, if it is a glue bullet cut the top of the tube at the end, put the lid back on and sit the glue with the open end upwards in the glass dappen.

You are now ready to glue your tips to your nails. Take the tip for your thumb and place a dab of glue on the underside of the tip, only on the part of the tip that will be going on to your nail, use the extended part of the glue bullet to run this glue around the entire well area of the tip.

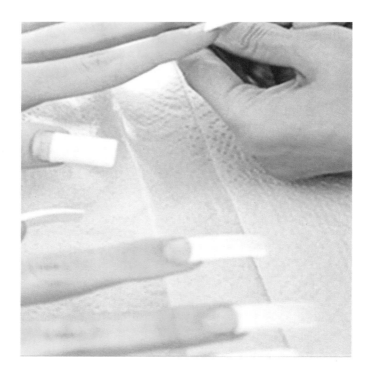

Place glue back into glass dappen and put the lid on. Take the tip, hold it at a 45 degree angle ---\ to the free edge of your nail, butt the inner edge of the tips well against the free edge of your nail and angle the tip down onto your nail, making sure the tip is on straight and not overhanging the cuticles on the side of your nail. Hold in place for about 10 seconds or until the glue has dried and the nail tip does not move.

Take your tip cutters and trim the tip to the desired size. Repeat this process for all your nails. Take your whiteblock and buff the shine off the tips to give a roughened surface, this is done to help the acrylic adhere to the tip.

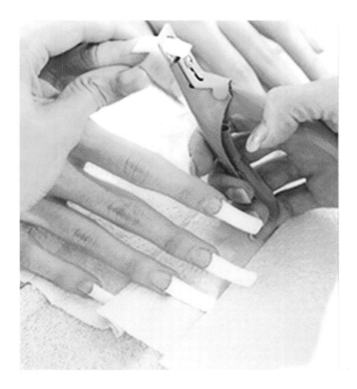

Chapter 3

APPLYING THE ACRYLIC

Many tips and hints and we will show two different methods of applying acrylic.

Section 1

1. The consistency

2. First stages of Application

3. Applying the Acrylic

4. Reverse Application Technique

5. Zone Application Technique

Make sure you have worked out the consistency ratios for your powders and monomer. You should have conditioned your application brush before starting.

At this stage you have done the following:

1. Buffed the shine off your nails with the whiteblock

2. Sized and applied the tips to your nails.

3. Cut your tips to the desired length.

4. Sprayed your nails again with Anti-Bac Solution

5. Brushed away excess dust from your nails.

Do one hand at a time, by this I mean doing the nails on one hand thoroughly, then repeating the processes again on the other hand. Use the products in the order listed below.

NAIL PREP

Nail Prep temporarily removes excess oils from the nail plate and this helps with adhesion of the acrylic. Put a small dab of Nail Prep onto each nail only where the natural nail is showing, let it dry thoroughly.

PRIMER

Primer is an acid and it sets down a chemical base for your application to adhere to. You only need one small dab of primer in the middle of each nail, the primer will spread to cover the natural nail plate. Be careful not to over apply this product because it is an acid it will sting if you have damaged cuticle or cuts in your cuticles. If this happens, try to ride it out until the stinging stops (usually less than 2 minutes). Let this dry thoroughly, many Primers look chalky when they are dry. It is imperative that this product has dried because if it hasn't you may end up contaminating your monomer with it by way of the brush.

You are now ready to start applying the acrylic. I will show you how to apply it through two different methods, one we will call Reverse and the other Zone. Have a practice with both methods and see which one suits you the best.

GETTING THE CONSISTENCY RIGHT

Pour some monomer into a dappen dish, dip your brush in and wipe the brush on the dappen to remove the excess liquid then put the tip of the brush onto the top of your powder and pull the brush towards you to pick up a bead, don't dip your brush into the powder vertically and then pull it out, doing this will give you a bead that is too big for the amount of liquid held in the brush and some of the powder will remain untouched by the monomer.

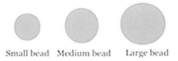
Small bead   Medium bead   Large bead

Draw circles the same size as above on a piece of paper and practice getting your liquid to ratio correct. Using a small amount of liquid by wiping lot of excess liquid from the brush, pick up a small bead of powder, wait until the powder has been consumed by the liquid (you will see this happening and make sure there is no powder on the brush that has not been touched by liquid) and place it in the centre of the first circle, watch how it spreads, if it spreads quickly and beyond the circle you have too much liquid, use less liquid. Do the same with the medium bead using a little more liquid than you did with the small bead. Keep practicing and you will get it right.

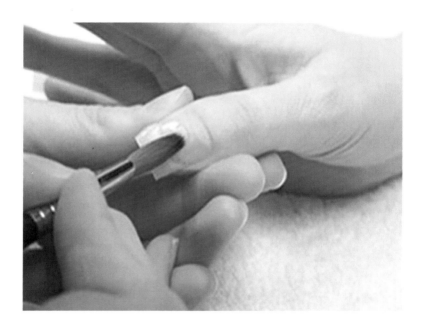

APPLYING ACRYLIC ON TO YOUR NAIL

When you are applying the acrylic onto your nail NEVER pull it down the nail with your brush, always PUSH the acrylic into place and pat gently on the top to smooth out ridges. A good quality acrylic powder and monomer will self level and only need a little pushing from you to get it into place. Do not apply it like nail polish as this will form ridges in the final product. Your acrylic consistency should seep slightly when applied to the nail, if it seeps too much you have too much liquid, if there is no movement you do not have enough liquid – practice again to get it right.

Section 2

Applying the Acrylic

Reverse Application Technique

On the diagram we have coloured the area we want to apply the acrylic to in pink. See how the acrylic is away from the cuticles at the sides and bottom of the nail.

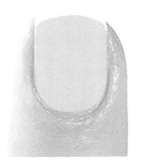

If you get acrylic on the cuticle when applying it to the nail, use an orangewood stick to run around nail between the acrylic and the cuticle to remove the acrylic from the cuticle. Do this while the acrylic is still wet. If the acrylic dries on the cuticle area you will need to file it off with a foam file.

Step 1

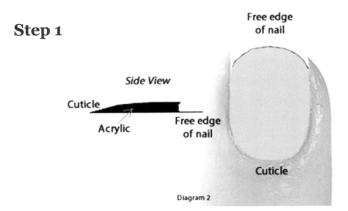

Looking at the diagram above, the pink area is where the first application of acrylic is going. Apply the first application of acrylic ending just over the attached edge of the tip, you can probably bring the acrylic down about 1 mm over this edge, using the sides of your brush, shape the acrylic into a curve (as shown in diagram 2) with your brush, push it into place and run your brush around the free edge area in a curve.

At this stage you are not taking the acrylic right to the edge of the tip, you are taking it just over the tip seam on the nail and at the same time not thinning the acrylic down by pushing it down to a thinner layer. This layer will help form part of the arch on the application (see page 32).

Don't worry if your smile line (the curve) is not perfect. Let the acrylic thoroughly dry.

The trick here is to get a file that has grit to the edges of that file and is a thin file. A Gold file for natural nails is perfect for this or a diamond metal file (most chemists stock these). With the file, file around that area to form a curve. Look at the side view on diagram 2 and you will see that you have a deeper ridge near the free edge where you have filed compared to the cuticle edge.

This smile line can be any type of curve you want.

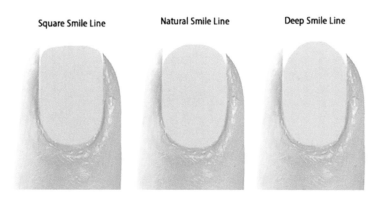

Square Smile Line   Natural Smile Line   Deep Smile Line

The different styles are achieved by the way you shape the edge of the acrylic with your brush and filing.

Step 2:

Once you are happy with the shape of your smile line you can now apply acrylic to the tip area. Here you are going to butt the acrylic up to the smile line area. Use the same process of acrylic application and place the bead in the centre of the tip. Gently push and press the acrylic into place, making sure you get acrylic up into the sides of the smile line and butting up against the first acrylic application. Follow the steps for forming the arch by blending the acrylic down so it is thinner at the free edge.

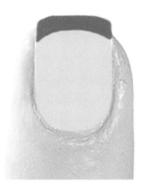

Don't worry if you get acrylic over the top of your first application and it looks like your smile line has disappeared, this can be filed down and it will bring back the clean smile line.

Check that the acrylic is dry.

ADDING NAIL ART WITH REVERSE APPLICATION

If you want to add nail art or embeds into your application, step 2 is the time to do this.

Next step is a third bead of acrylic and this is placed on the centre of the entire nail, including the tip.

Press the acrylic into place with the sides and body of your brush. The aim with this layer is the form an arch, if you haven't already done this and carry the acrylic over the seam area where the tip is adhered to the nail to give it strength. With this layer you also need to press the acrylic down on an angle towards the free edge of the tip, like you did at the cuticle area. Again, if it is too thick you can file it down to the desired thickness. With this third bead try to blend it in on the edges with the previous applications, once it is dry you can also blend it in with a file or whiteblock after it is dry.

When the acrylic is totally dry use a whiteblock to buff down the acrylic and remove any brush marks or ridges that may have formed. Remember to keep the shape of the arch in the nail and buff down from the centre of the nail to the cuticles and the free edge.

Using a black foam file, file and shape the free edge of the tip and file underneath the tip to remove any bits of acrylic that may have flowed over the edge at application.

When you are happy with the finished nail, take a grey buffing block and buff over the entire nail area to obtain a smooth finish.

At this point your acrylic may look cloudy. This look will disappear when you apply a top coat to seal the acrylic. If you are worried about any lines of the tip seam showing you can wet the tip slightly with a little water when it is dry and this will show how the finished tip will look when you apply the top coat. If you do have ridges showing this can be hidden with nail art and corrected the next time you re balance your acrylic. If you do not want to use nail art then you will need to file the acrylic back to file down the seam or lines. While starting out you can lightly moisten each application layer as you go, but do not apply the next layer until the first is totally dry if you moistened it with a little water.

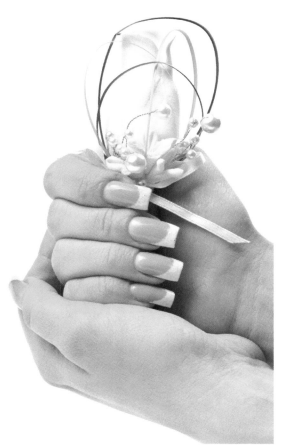

Add a shimmer finish to your final layer of acrylic by mixing a tiny bit of opal glitter to your acrylic powder. Use a ratio of 6 parts powder to 1 part glitter.

ORIGINAL ACRYLIC APPLICATION TECHNIQUE
ZONE METHOD

Start with the first medium bead as described previously, but this time do not take it over the seam line of the tip, split the nail area into 3 zones.

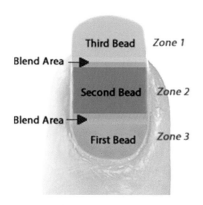

Apply the first bead and blend it into the second bead area a little.

Apply the second bead starting slightly above the lower blend of the first bead and blend the lower part of the second bead into zone 1.

Apply the third bead and blend it into Zone 2.

Forming the Arch

When you are applying the acrylic you will also need to form the arch in the centre of the nail, when you place the first bead in the centre of the zone you are working in, use your brush to gently push the acrylic towards the sides of the nail leaving it slightly higher in the centre to form the arch, blend the acrylic down to the cuticle area around the nail the free edge (see the diagram above). This can be formed with the second application of acrylic.

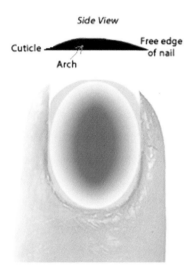

When the acrylic is dry you can add another thin layer of acrylic over the entire nail area or if you think the first layer applied using the beads is ample and will be strong enough you can file the sides of the nail and free edge of the nail to shape, then follow with a buff using a whiteblock and finally a buff with a grey buffer to smooth the application.

When you are happy with the shape apply nail polish top coat to the nails.

If you find that you did not pick up enough mix to cover an area you can fix this by applying another small bead to the missed area and blending it in. As in the Reverse Application Technique you will also have to form the nail arch.

FINISHING UP

The most important thing now is to clean up:

- Get some paper towels and fold them over 2-3 times. Take your brush and hold it in Brush Cleaner solution for a minute, only put the bristles into the solution, do not submerge the metal part of the brush, remove and wipe the brush over the paper towels. Repeat and when you remove the brush this time place the bristles down on the paper towel and using a cuticle stick gently use the bevelled edge to scrape inside the bristles from the top of the bristles to the end to loosen up any acrylic stuck in there. Pop the brush back into the brush cleaner again for a minute, remove and wipe again, check with the cuticle stick to make sure there is no acrylic hiding in the bristles. DO NOT sandwich the bristles between layers of paper and pull as this will eventually ruin your brush by loosening the bristles.

- Using Antibacterial solution give your files and buffers a gentle spray all over, don't saturate them. Set aside to try.

- If you have any monomer left over do not throw it down the sink, grab an absorbent paper towel, scrunch it up and push it into the dappen to absorb the liquid, place this in a plastic bag, seal and dispose of it in the bin.

- If you used a towel on your table while doing your nails, take it and shake it outside to minimise dust in your work area or home.

- Make sure the lid on your glue is on tight because it will dry out very quickly.

- When your files are dry pop them into a plastic bag to keep them clean, do not seal the bag just in case there is still some moisture on them.

- Buy a large plastic box to keep all your nail equipment in.

SMOOTHEAZE FORMS / DUAL FORMS

Another option for applying acrylic if you are finding it difficult to get a smooth consistent finish. After about a minute tap the form with your brush and if it sounds hollow lift it off, the acrylic application underneath will have a beautiful shine and you will not need to do any filing on the surface, only on the sides to clean up.

These forms do need replacing after every 5-6 uses if you want to keep getting the shine. The underneath surface starts to diminish slightly with use but if you are happy to apply a top coat.

Application Instructions for Smootheaze Nail Forms

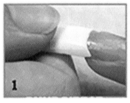

Apply tip to free eage of nail.

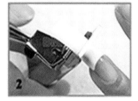

Trim tip to desired length.

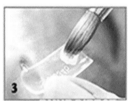

Pick up bead of acrylic powder as you would normally with your brush.

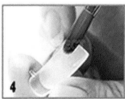

Fill your form with the acrylic beads. Enusre there is enough to form arch.

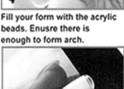

File edges of tip after form is removed.

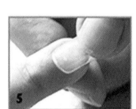

Press form firmly onto nail starting at 45 degree angle from top to free edge, hold.

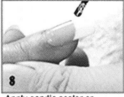

Apply acrylic sealer or top coat

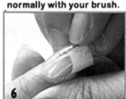

Hold for 20 secs, leave form in place, do other nails then remove by lifting off.

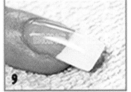

ENJOY!

Other types of forms available are square and horseshoe shape. These are made of strong shiny paper and can be molded to fit each individual nail. These are used to form the tip with acrylic instead of applying a tip. The acrylic is adhered to the natural nail. Using forms allows the flexibility to create different shaped tips.

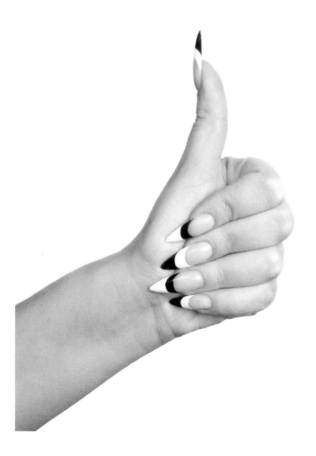

Try a two tone French nail effect. Use the Reverse Application technique and butt up 3 colours instead of two.

These tips are called European Cusp tips. This style can also be created using paper forms.

Chapter 4

REBALANCING & REFILLING

After a few weeks your nails will have grown and you will need to refill and if you have french tips you will need to rebalance these.

After a couple of weeks you will notice that the acrylic application is starting to move down the nail as your nail grows out, if it is only minimal then you can apply a fresh coat of top coat and this will keep you out of trouble for a while. If the distance between your cuticle and the edge that was blended at the cuticle is becoming very noticeable or there is lifting it is time to refill that area.

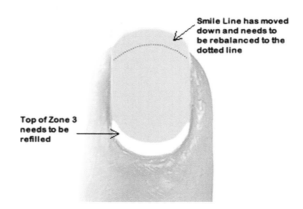

Smile Line has moved down and needs to be rebalanced to the dotted line

Top of Zone 3 needs to be refilled

Before you start, spray your hands and nails with anti-bac solution.

REFILLING

If you are getting lifting at the cuticle area you will need to cut this back with cuticle nippers to where there is no lifting or you can blend carefully with a file without touching the natural nail.

With a black foam file, file over the top of the acrylic to remove some of the acrylic (at least a layer). Do not file it all off, leave at least one layer there.

Using a manicure brush, brush away the dust from the nail and cuticle areas.

TAKE CARE when applying the primer that you do not get any on the acrylic remaining on the nail as this could make the acrylic go yellow.

Take a small bead of acrylic and apply it to the centre of the refill area and using your brush push it in to place taking care to blend it at the cuticle edge and over the existing acrylic. Another option is to use two small beads placing the first one off centre and blending to one side and half of the refill area and another small bead to do the other side. When the acrylic is dry, using a black foam file or if your blend is not high use a whiteblock, file or buff over the blended area to blend it in well with the old acrylic.

Now you can apply another thinner layer of acrylic over the entire nail area. Remember to keep the arch in place as well when you are pushing the acrylic into place.

REBALANCING

Using a black foam file remove the acrylic from the tip area and back to where you want the smile line to be, do this by filing down on the top and filing in a way to create a new smile line. Then file down a layer on the remainder of the acrylic on the nail. When you have got the acrylic off, use a file to the vertical edge of the old acrylic to file in a new line, in the same way you did when you first created the original line. Using white powder and liquid take a medium bead of powder/liquid and apply off the centre of the nail, butt this up to the smile line, push into place at the free edge sides of the tip and do not panic if white goes on to the existing acrylic because you can quickly file this back down when it is dry. If you have white tips on, continue as above and fill with white powder to the smile line. Go over the entire area with a whiteblock to smooth out any bumps or ridges.

Apply a thin layer of acrylic using 2-3 medium beads, pushing it into place with your brush and keeping the arch in place. Buff the entire area down with a whiteblock making sure to keep the arch looking nice and in the right place and to remove any ridges or lumps. Finish with nail polish top coat.

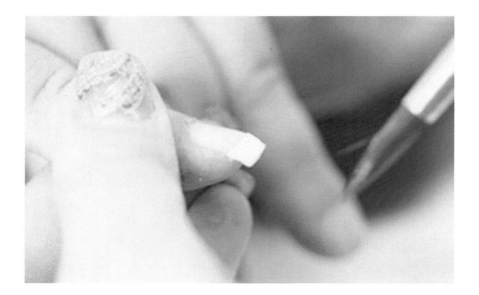

Section 2

MAINTAINING YOUR NAILS

MANICURE

Every day apply a little cuticle oil to your cuticles and rub it in well. This will help keep your cuticles soft and assist to minimise lifting.

Once a week gently push back the cuticles using an orangewood stick on the bevelled edge or a cuticle pusher.

Once a week remove the polish top coat, if you have used one and reapply, this will help keep the nails looking fresh and it will also give you a chance to see if there is any lifting.

If there is lifting try to fix it as soon as possible to avoid any chance of bacteria getting into that area.

Treat your nails gently. If you knock a nail badly and believe there is bleeding under the nail, remove the acrylic immediately, if you cannot do this yourself, go to an experienced manicurist and get them to do it for you.

If you rip an acrylic nail it can rip your natural nail, again if you cannot remove it yourself go to a professional.

REMOVING ACRYLIC

Removing acrylic takes a little time and needs to be done properly. Unless you are a trained professional do not use an electric drill to remove the acrylic. You will need the following:

- Soak Off

- black foam files varying in grit from 100 to 180 or 240

- cuticle sticks

- soaking trays or cotton wool and aluminum foil

- white block

- grey buffing block

- cuticle oil

Start by filing off as much acrylic as you can with the coarsest grit file. Be very careful not to file your cuticles and cut them.

Then fill your soak trays with Soak Off solution and hold your fingers in for about 30 mins. If you do not have soak off trays, saturate some cotton wool balls with soak off, place the soaked cotton wool over the nail and wrap with aluminum foil to hold the cotton wool in placed and stop the soak off solution leaking out.

After 30 mins check your nails, grab an orangewood stick and with the bevelled edge remove the soft acrylic by pushing it off the nail. Keep repeating this process until you have all the acrylic off. If you are unable to soak it all off, get it down as close to the natural nail as possible.

If you still have a thin layer of acrylic left, use the grey buffing block on the sanding side and gently buff away the remainder of the acrylic. Be careful not to file down onto the natural nail because this will damage the nail plate. DO NOT pick the acrylic off because this will rip away a layer or two of natural nail and damage your nail. The idea is to get the acrylic off without damaging your natural nail. Damage to the natural nail plate can let in infections and make it difficult for future acrylic nails to be applied.

When you have removed your acrylics your nails will probably be a little soft, leave your nails for about a week, applying cuticle oil every day to help strengthen them. If they are still soft or weak after a week, please do not be tempted to reapply acrylic because doing will cause further damage in the long run.

Chapter 5

NAIL ART

Nail art application on acrylic nails is endless with all the options available to the budding nail artist.

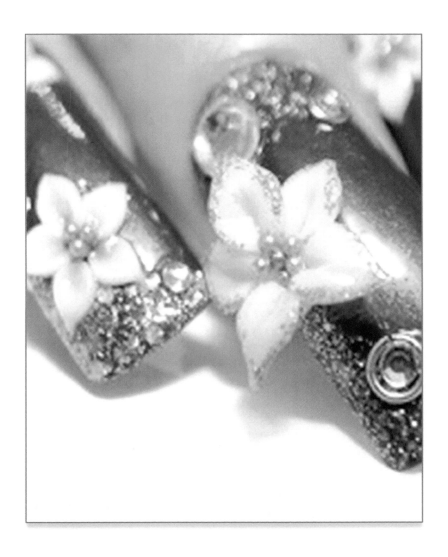

There are many different mediums you can use for nail art, how you use them is entirely up to your imagination, look around the internet for photos and inspiration.

GLITTER

There are several different types of glitter - superfine, fine, shapes and chunky. Glitter can be mixed in with acrylic powder at a ratio of 5 parts powder and 2 parts glitter. Mix the powder and glitter in a separate dappen dish, load the brush with liquid and pick up the size bead you need, you work it the same way as you would if it was just acrylic powder. Glitter is fantastic for creating sparkling french nails

FLITTER GLITTER

This is a name we gave to a glitter type product that is small strands of multi colours. These are added to acrylic powder in the same way glitter is.

Mylar

This is shell type product with a hologram effect, it comes in a range of colours and looks amazing when the light catches it. It is chunky, to adhere it to the nail dab on a little nail glue to the area and using a moistened end of a toothpick pick up a small piece of the mylar and set it down on your glued area.

COLOURED ACRYLIC POWDER

Coloured acrylic powder is readily available and can be used to create french tips or used to create designs in acrylic which is applied as the first layer. It is applied the same way as normal acrylic. We recommend applying a thin layer of clear acrylic over the top of coloured acrylic applications.

Another way to achieve coloured acrylic is with coloured monomer. There are liquid concentrates available which are added to the monomer, only a small amount is needed. Once the colour is mixed with the liquid in the dappen, load the brush with liquid and then pick up a bead of clear powder for a translucent look and apply as normal. For an opaque colour use white powder. With the liquids you can also mix the colours together to create even more colours.

Other nail art products that can be embedded into acrylic are:

- laser strands
- foil chips
- nail art foil
- bullion
- spangles
- striping tape

A set of nail art brushes is always handy to have, get a good set with 7-15 brushes. Some nail art paints can be used on the first application of acrylic and the second layer of acrylic gently patted down on top of the nail art paint. Try dry brushing nail art paint with a fan brush from one side of the nail to the other, this will create a tiger effect. Using the fan brush pick up some paint on the edge of the brush, wipe it on a paper towel and with the remainder of paint on the brush start at the side edge of your nail and pull the brush across, the paint will lessen as the brush goes across the nail and give thinner lines towards the other side of the nail. Don't hestiate to experiment with colours either, using a little imagination your nail art design gallery will become endless.

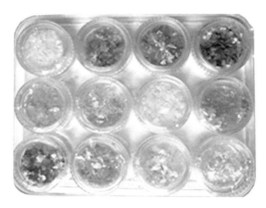

Mylar which usually has a hologram effect and is made from shell.

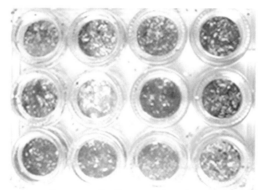

Diamond shape mylar made from plastic or metal and has a hologram effect

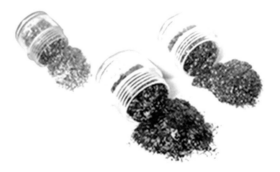

Flitter Glitter is a string glitters with a hologram effect. Add 1 part of flitter to 4 parts of acrylic powder.

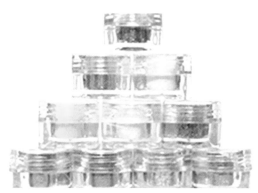

Glitter is fantastic for mixing in acrylic or your topcoat, use it with other nail art as well. Use at the ratio of 3 parts acrylic powder to 1 part glitter

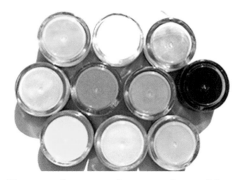

Coloured Acrylic powders can be purchased in sets or individually, use then as you would normal acrylic powder.

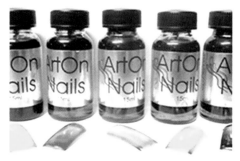

Colour Concentrate is a liquid you can add to monomer or gel, using one drop at a time, use with clear powder for a translucent look or white powder for a pastel opaque look.

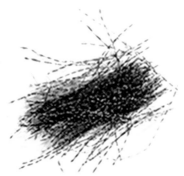

Laser Strips can be embedded into acrylic and give a hologram effect. There is a variety of colours available.

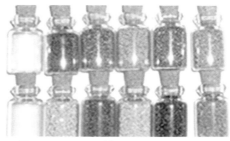

Bullion beads offer a 3D effect when embedded Into acrylic. These can be glued on individually to create lines and shapes of mixed in with your acrylic mix, but doing it this way will mean you will need to apply a slightly thicker layer of acrylic to ensure the beads are covered and not exposed so they are not filed down.

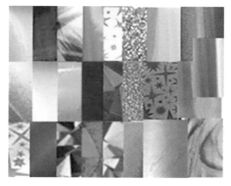

Foil transfer paper can be used as an embed on the first acrylic application or on top of the finished nail.

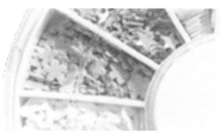

Spangles are available in many different colours and shapes; embed these on the first acrylic layer, most have a hologram effect. They are small plastic shapes.

Nail Art ideas can be found in any craft shop, just look for small items. Acrylic Paints can also be used, and a good nail art brush set always comes in handy.

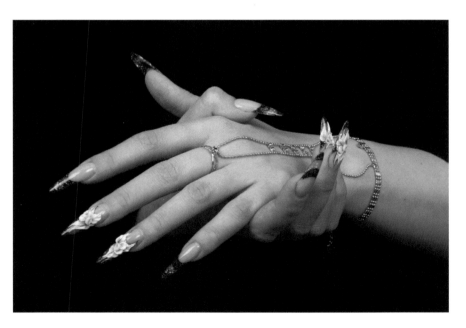

You can also create flowers with acrylic as well by using a small bead of acrylic, place the bead on your nail and put the point of your brush into on the edge, holding your brush over the bead, gently lay the brush, from the pointed end, back into the acrylic, this will spread it a little to look like a petal.

NAIL ART TECHNIQUES WITH ACRYLIC

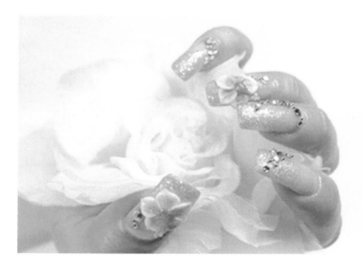

The effect on these nails is achieved by using two glitter colours. Apply the darker colour on the free edge of the tip up about 1/3rd of the nail, then apply the lighter colour glitter blending it in with to the darker colour and up the next 1/3rd of the nail. Apply another thin layer of acrylic over the entire nail area and buff down. The flowers on the nails are created using acrylic, these can also be bought separately and there are molds available that are specifically for creating acrylic flowers and shapes to be put on the nail. The flowers are glued on before the final layer of acrylic and the final layer helps to set them in. Rhinestones have also been added to the final nail with glue and then the entire nail finished with top coat.

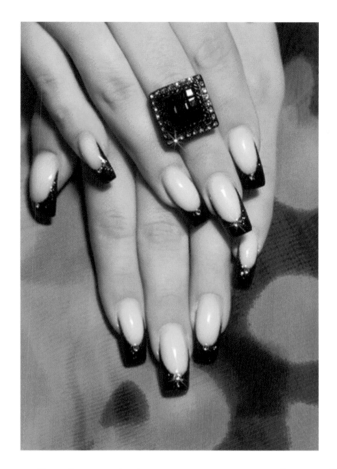

Reverse application technique creates a stunning smile line. A Pink Cover Acrylic powder has been used; this is an opaque colour, over the natural nail area. Black coloured acrylic powder is used to create the french nail finish and to this glitter has been added. Another way to get glitter on is to dab glitter on to the wet acrylic with your brush and it will set into the acrylic as it dries.

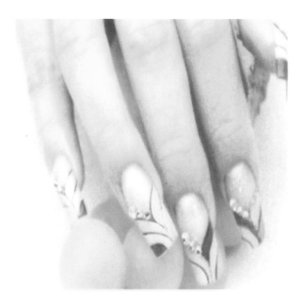

This design is easily done by butting up acrylic colours using small beads, start with the reverse acrylic application technique and file back the acrylic at the smile line to start the design, leave a small gap between each colour and fill this with a dark colour acrylic. If it goes over the other coloured acrylic, it doesn't matter because it can be buffed back to reveal the design. Rhinestones have been glued on to the top and then two coats of topcoat to finish. If you don't feel confident enough to do this with acrylic you can always finish your nails and then use acrylic nail art paints to paint the design on. Finish with a nail art top coat to seal the paint.

AIRBRUSHED NAIL TIPS OR DESIGNED TIPS

The easiest way to do nail art is with predesigned tips, they can look like a painted design or a solid colour. They are applied to the nail the same way a normal tip is applied, but one thing you need to be careful of is buffing the tip down for acrylic, some tips you can and some when you try to buff down loose the design. Before you glue them to your nail test a tip in a size that you will use the least of, buff half the tip down and then apply acrylic to the entire tip, check to make sure that the buff did not remove the design and that where the tip is not buffed that the acrylic adhered to the tip.

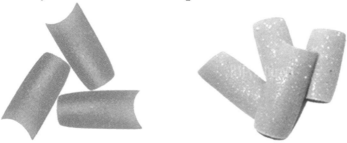

Glitter Tips are a pre designed tip with glitter glued on to the tip, all you need to do is glue the tip on and apply the acrylic as normal.

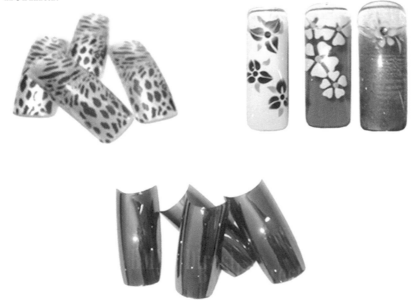

Always do a test on a airbrushed or coloured tips before gluing them on. Test to see if the tips can be buffed down before applying the acrylic or that they will take the acrylic without buffing.

Chapter 6

TROUBLESHOOTING

Sometimes things can go wrong, hopefully here we can give you the answers to any issues you may have.

If you are having trouble with natural nails or lifting, hopefully the following will help you drill down to find out the cause.

PROBLEM NAILS
Ever wondered why you are asked to remove nail polish before you go into hospital, it is because nails tell a lot about a person's health.

WHY ARE MY NAILS YELLOW?
This can be caused by nail polish staining your nails, smoking, household cleaners, etc. There are yellow out polishes available and they put a bluish colour over the nail to hide the yellow but do not get rid of the yellowing. When cleaning or using chemicals wear gloves to protect your nails.

MY NAILS KEEP BREAKING.
Any number of things can cause this and to find the cause it is an elimination process, these are some of the things you should look at:
- a mineral deficiency
- bad filing technique on the natural nail, never file backwards and forwards, always file the natural nail in one direction only.
- Hereditary
- household chemicals
- medication

Nails splitting and peeling can be caused by a mineral deficiency as well.

CUTICLES ARE SPLITTING
This can be painful, using cuticle nippers, very carefully to nip off the offending piece of cuticle, do not cut into cuticle that is not loose. Keep your hands clean if it bleeds to avoid any infection getting in. Using cuticle oils or hand cream on a regular basis will help keep your cuticles soft and remember to use gloves when doing work that is hard on your hands.

WHITE SPOTS ON MY NAILS
These appear when your diet is lacking either in some of all of these elements - calcium, zinc or iron. Try adding these one at time to see which one it is.

SORE NAILS
If your nails feel sore or itchy you may have a fungal infection, remove your acrylic nails immediately and seek medication advise. Do not leave it because by leaving it you will end up damaging your nails and if this happens chances are you will not be able to wear acrylics or any type of artificial nails again.

ACRYLICS LIFTING
There are a number of variables that can cause acrylic nails to lift and again you will have to go through the process of elimination to find out what the cause is.

An incorrect tip size has been used - the tip was too small and has been forced to sit down on the nail against the tips natural shape. If you have a nail that seems to be in between tip sizes, use the bigger tip and file it down at the side to make it smaller to ensure that the well of the tip that will sit on the natural nail sits neatly and does not have to be forced down to sit flush with the nail. A tip that has been forced will eventually tear away from the glue and start to lift.

A lot of lifting problems stem from the prep process right at the start not being done properly.
- natural oils not being removed with prep.

- natural nail not being buffed down to remove the shine
- cuticle not being pushed back therefore acrylic is sitting on the pterygium (cuticle over growth) and not the nail.
- dust not being brushed away from the nail before starting application.
- nails are moist
- they need to be totally dry.
- misuse of nails
- knocking nails, typing, banging etc.
- diseased nail plate.
- biting or picking at the nails.

Other things that can cause lifting:
- medication that you are taking.
- Allergy to the product itself.
- bacteria in your system.

Processes in Application that may cause lifting:
- Contaminated Primer - dust may have gotten into your primer.
- mixing products from different manufacturer's, some products just do not go together and are incompatible.
- the natural nail area has been saturated with too much primer. You only need to use one dab and the primer will spread, do not apply anything else until it is totally dry.

If you are using a good quality acrylic and monomer and experience lifting it can generally be attributed to one of the above causes and not the product.

INFECTIONS
We cannot stress enough as to how important it is that you keep your equipment clean, make sure your files and buffers are sprayed with anti-bac and clean for the next time. If you get an infection see a Doctor immediately.

CPSIA information can be obtained at www.ICGtesting.com
Printed in the USA
LVIW01n1718030116
468890LV00002B/33

* 9 7 8 0 6 4 6 5 8 8 2 6 1 *